OPTIMIZE YOUR HEALTH

A Comprehensive Guide to Fitness, Diet, and Nutrition

Jennifer Chimdia

Optimize your health

Copyright © 2024 Jennifer Chimdia

ISBN:9798321386354

DEDICATION

Grateful to God and to my husband for the unwavering love and encouragement through this journey

CONTENTS

ACKNOWLEDGMENTS

Grateful for insights to optimize health and well-being journey

1 INTRODUCTION

Achieving optimal health and fitness is a journey toward physical, mental, and emotional well-being. It involves adopting habits that promote vitality, strength, and resilience. From nourishing the body with nutritious foods to engaging in regular physical activity, every choice plays a crucial role in shaping our overall wellness. By prioritizing healthy habits and embracing a balanced lifestyle, individuals can enhance their quality of life and unlock their full potential for vitality and longevity.

It's very important to note that Health and fitness are crucial for overall well-being. They enhance physical strength, mental resilience, and emotional balance, reducing the risk of various diseases and promoting longevity. Additionally, they improve productivity, boost self-esteem, and foster a positive outlook on life. Regular exercise and a balanced diet contribute to better sleep, sharper cognitive function, and a higher quality of life, allowing individuals to fully engage in daily activities and pursue their goals with vigor.

Most importantly understanding the major goals for achieving a healthy lifestyle is very crucial which includes

1. Nutrition: Minimize the intake of processed food and focus more on fruits vegetables, lean protein and whole meals.

2.Physical Exercise: Daily exercise like walking a distance, jogging, swimming etc can be very helpful in achieving a healthy lifestyle. It's very important to get a time goal for it

3.Bed Rest: It's very important to have at least 8 hours of sleep at night.

4.Stress Control: Take charge of your daily activities and develop some strategies on how to reduce stress such as doing what makes you happy.

5.Hydration: Always remember to take enough water based on your individual needs.

6.Social Interaction: Spend quality time with family and friends.

7.Screen Time: Set limits on screen time for activities like watching TV, using smart phones, or browsing the internet, and allocate more time for activities that promote well-being.

8.Medical Checkup: Schedule regular appointments with your doctor

2

RUDIMENTARY OF NUTRITION AND BALANCE DIET

This involves consuming a wide variety of foods in the right proportions, thereby providing the essential nutrients for a healthy lifestyle and longevity.

This includes the macro nutrients (fats, protein, carbohydrates)and the micronutrients (vitamins and minerals)

IMPORTANCE OF THE MACRO AND MICRO NUTRIENTS.

Carbohydrate: Carbohydrates are very important as they provide the body with its main source of energy, fueling essential bodily functions and enabling optimal physical activities.

Protein: Proteins are crucial for building tissues, repairing worn out tissues, supporting immunity and serving as enzymes.

Fat: Fats are essential for energy storage, hormone production, absorption of fat-soluble vitamins, insulation, and maintaining cell structure and function.

Vitamin: They help in metabolism, immune support healthy bone and vision.

It's important to understand the relationship between calories balance and its impact on weight management.

Calorie balance refers to the equilibrium between calories consumed and expended. To manage weight, maintaining a balance by controlling intake and increasing expenditure is crucial for achieving desired outcomes

How To Establish Principle Of A Balanced Diet

Establishing a principle of a balanced diet incorporating whole foods, vegetables, and fruits .Begin by understanding the importance of each food group: whole grains provide fiber and essential nutrients, lean proteins support repair of and build up of tissue, healthy fats aid in nutrient absorption while vegetables and fruits offer vitamins and minerals.

Plan meals around these components, emphasizing variety and diversity. Incorporate a rainbow of fruits and vegetables to ensure a wide array of nutrients and phytochemical. Prioritize whole, minimally processed foods over refined options, opting for whole-grain bread, pasta, and cereals. Include a source of lean protein like chicken and fish.

Balance portion sizes to meet individual energy needs and maintain a healthy weight and always remember to stay hydrated.

Most importantly, Be mindful your eating practices by paying attention to hunger and fullness cues.

To Maintain a balanced diet, one must prioritize taking whole foods, including vegetables and fruits, proteins and healthy fats and avoid being dehydrated

3

EXERCISE AND FITNESS ROUTINE

Exercise is any physical activity done to improve health and fitness.

It comprises of wide range of activities including cardiovascular activities like running and jogging etc.

Exercise is vital for physical and mental well-being. It strengthens the heart and muscles, boosts metabolism, and helps in weight management.

Exercise releases endorphins, reducing stress and anxiety, and constant exercise also promotes longevity.

Types Of Exercise

There are various types of exercise to optimize a healthy lifestyle.

Aerobic exercise; This includes swimming, running and they said to improve cardiovascular health.

Strength training such as weight lifting, aids in metabolism

Flexibility exercises like stretching and yoga.

Balance exercises; This enhances stability such as standing on one leg.

Common Exercise Barriers

The common Exercise Barriers include lack of time, motivation, knowledge, and access to facilities.

To overcome these barriers:

1.Time: Schedule workouts like appointments and prioritize exercise.

2.Motivation: Set specific, achievable goals, find enjoyable activities, exercise with a friend, relative, spouse or colleague for accountability, and vary your routine to keep it more interesting.

3.Knowledge: Seek guidance from a professional/ trainer, start with simple exercises, and educate yourself through reliable sources.

4.Access: Explore affordable options like home workouts, outdoor activities, or online fitness programs. Utilize community centers and parks.

By addressing these barriers systematically and with determination, individuals can establish a consistent exercise routine that aligns with their lifestyle and goals.

Setting Fitness Goals Based on Individual Needs

To set goals based on individual needs, and assess personal desires, abilities, and limitations. Create specific, measurable, achievable, relevant, and time-bound (SMART) goals.
Tailor goals to match individual preferences, such as weight loss, strength gain, flexibility improvement etc.

How To Incorporate Variety and Progression To Keep Work Out Challenging And Effective

Gradually increase intensity, and duration to continually challenge the body and promote growth.

Engage in new activities like swimming, yoga, hiking etc.

By consistently introducing and engaging in variety and progression, individuals can sustain motivation, and avoid stagnation thereby maximizing fitness gains over time

4

SLEEP; IS A MAJOR THERAPY TO COMBAT STRESS.

Sleep is vital for stress management as it allows the body and mind to recover for several hours every night, In this process the eyes are closed, muscles are relaxed and consciousness of the environment is suspended.

The quality of sleep required varies on an individual depending on the age.

Adequate sleep enhances resilience to stress, promotes mental clarity, fosters emotional stability, improves memories, and enhances learning and problem-solving skills contributing to overall well-being and stress reduction.

How To Improve Sleep

1.Establish a consistent sleep schedule, going to bed and waking up at the same time every day.

2. Limit exposure to screens, especially blue light, before bedtime.

3. Ensure your sleep environment is conducive to rest, with a comfortable mattress and pillow.

4. Avoid consuming stimulants like caffeine and heavy meals close to bedtime.

5. Incorporate regular exercise into your routine, but avoid vigorous activity close to bedtime.

7. Manage stress through relaxation techniques such as breathing exercises.

8. Limit daytime naps to avoid disrupting

nighttime sleep patterns.

9. Seek professional help if sleep problems persist

5

ADOPTING ECO-CONSCIOUS DAILY PRACTICES FOR HOLISTIC WELL-BEING.

Adopting eco-conscious daily practices for holistic well-being involves integrating environmentally friendly habits into every aspect of life. This includes reducing waste by recycling and composting, conserving energy and water, and choosing sustainable products. By prioritizing these practices, individuals contribute to environmental preservation while also enhancing their well-being. Eating locally sourced and organic foods supports both personal health and sustainable agriculture. Engaging in activities such as walking or cycling instead of driving reduces carbon emissions and promotes physical fitness. Ultimately, this holistic approach fosters a sense of connection to the planet and promotes a healthier lifestyle for individuals and the environment alike.

Strategies for cultivating healthy eating, consistent physical activity, and mindful self-care routines.

This involves a multifaceted approach. Begin by setting realistic and achievable goals tailored to your lifestyle and preferences. Prioritize whole foods rich in nutrients, incorporating diverse fruits, vegetables, lean proteins, and whole grains into meals. Schedule regular physical activity sessions, choosing activities you enjoy to enhance adherence. Practice mindfulness and stress management techniques such as meditation or deep breathing exercises to promote mental well-being. Ensure adequate sleep to support overall health and recovery. Lastly, maintain a balanced approach, allowing flexibility and occasional indulgences while staying committed to long-term well-being goals

6

DIETARY SUPPLEMENTS AND THEIR FUNCTIONS

"Dietary supplements and their functions" refer to products taken orally that contain one or more dietary ingredients intended to supplement one's diet and provide specific health benefits. These supplements include vitamins, amino acids, vitamins and herbs.

Nutritional supplements include:

1.   Multivitamins: A blend of vitamin blend of essential vitamins in a single supplement dose. Multivitamins contains

essential vitamins and minerals. They are designed to complement a healthy diet by providing nutrients that may be lacking. Multivitamins support various bodily functions, including metabolism, boost immunity, enhancing optimal health and vitality.

2. Omega-3 fatty acids: Derived from fish oil or plant sources like flaxseed, omega-3s support heart health, and brain function, and reduce inflammation.

3.Protein: Often derived from soy, pea, or other sources. Protein powder is commonly used by fitness enthusiasts and athletes to increase protein intake.

4.Calcium: Vital for bone health and muscle function, calcium supplements are commonly used, especially by those at risk of osteoporosis. Calcium It's found in dairy products, fortified foods and leafy greens. Calcium supplements are available for those who may not get enough from their diet, especially individuals at risk of osteoporosis.

5. Vitamin D: Vitamin D is a fat-soluble vitamin. It's synthesized in the skin upon exposure to sunlight and found in some foods like fatty fish and fortified dairy products. Vitamin D supports bone health, immune function, and mood regulation. Many people have low levels of vitamin D, especially in regions with limited sunlight.

6. Vitamin C: Vitamin C which is also known as ascorbic acid, is a water-soluble vitamin found in fruits and vegetables, particularly citrus fruits, strawberries, and bell peppers. It acts as an antioxidant, supporting immune function, collagen synthesis, wound healing, and iron absorption.

7. Magnesium: Supports muscle and nerve function, as well as bone health.

8. Iron: Essential for red blood cell formation and oxygen transport. Iron supplements are commonly used to prevent or treat iron deficiency anemia, especially among menstruating women and vegetarians.

9. Probiotics: These are live bacteria and yeasts that are good for your digestive system. They are often used to promote gut health and support digestion. They are commonly found in fermented foods like yogurt.
They support gut health by balancing the intestinal microbiota, aiding digestion, and boosting the immune system.

10. Coenzyme Q10 (CoQ10): Acts as an antioxidant and is involved in energy production within cells. It's commonly used to support heart health and as an energy booster.

It's necessary to note that while supplements can be beneficial for some individuals, they should not replace a balanced diet. Consulting with a healthcare professional before starting any supplement regimen is advised, especially for those with underlying health conditions or taking medications..

7

HOW TO DEFEAT SOME COMMON CHALLENGE AND PLATEAUS

To begin a journey toward a healthy life style and fitness is often filled with motivation. However, along the way, it's common to encounter challenges and plateaus that can discourage you and slow down your progress

WAYS TO OVERCOME CHALLENGES AND HANDLE PLATEAUS

1. Identify the most common challenges which includes:

Lack of motivation: Feeling demotivated or

uninspired can hinder progress. Always try to remain motivated

Time factor: Balancing your daily activities and responsibilities can make it challenging to prioritize exercise and healthy eating.

Stress eating: Using foods as a coping mechanism for stress or boredom can sabotage your efforts.

Illness: feeling unwell can disrupt your progress

2. Measures of Overcoming Challenges

Stay motivated and remind yourself of the reasons why you started your health journey.

Prioritize personal wellness: Create time for activities that nourish your body and soul, such as meditation, hobbies, or relaxation techniques.

Seek for support: Lean on friends or family for encouragement and accountability.

Celebrate your little effort to stay motivated and build momentum.

3. **Breaking Through Plateaus**.

Incorporate varieties into your workouts by trying new exercises .

Evaluate your dietary habits and make tweaks as needed, such as increasing protein intake, reducing portion sizes, or incorporating more Whole Foods. Limit the intake of processed foods.

Reassess your goals and set new challenges to keep your motivation levels high and push past stagnation.

Be patient and persistent

4. **Deal with Setbacks** .

Most importantly practice self-compassion and avoid self-criticism, recognizing that progress is not always linear. Stay focused on the bigger picture and remind yourself that setbacks are temporary obstacles on the path to long-term success.

By recognizing and addressing common challenges and plateaus head-on, you can navigate the ups and downs of your health and fitness journey with resilience and determination. Remember that setbacks are not a sign of failure but rather an opportunity for growth and transformation. Keep pushing forward, and you'll emerge stronger and more empowered than ever before.

8
CONCLUSION

Optimizing your health is a journey that requires commitment, but the rewards are immeasurable.

Optimize your health is a broad guide to achieving a holistic well-being, offering strategies for enhancing mental and physical vitality.

Start by prioritizing a balanced diet rich in fruits, vegetables, lean proteins, and whole grains.

It's very important to stay hydrated, aim for at least eight glasses of water a day. Consistent exercise is necessary.

Prioritize sleep; aim for 7-9 hours each night to allow your body to rest .
Manage stress effectively.

Additionally, prioritize regular medical check-ups with your doctor . Surround yourself with relatives, friends or colleagues that encourages your health goals. Remember, consistent steps can lead to significant improvement.

Implementing these practices will not only optimize your physical health but also enhance your mental and emotional well-being. Start today; your future self will thank you.

ABOUT THE AUTHOR

The author of "Optimize Your Health" is a seasoned wellness guru, offering expert guidance to enhance physical and mental well-being. Their book provides actionable strategies and insights to cultivate a balanced and vibrant lifestyle.

www.ingramcontent.com/pod-product-compliance
Lightning Source LLC
Chambersburg PA
CBHW051927250726
48659CB00002B/875